# HAND SANITIZER RECIPES

## HOW TO MAKE YOUR HAND SANITIZER FOR A VIRUS-FREE HOME

By
**CATALINA SMITH**

© Copyright 2020 by Catalina Smith
All rights reserved.

This document is geared towards providing exact and reliable information with regards to the topic and issue covered. The publication is sold with the idea that the publisher is not required to render accounting, officially permitted, or otherwise, qualified services. If advice is necessary, legal or professional, a practiced individual in the profession should be ordered.

- From a Declaration of Principles which was accepted and approved equally by a Committee of the American Bar Association and a Committee of Publishers and Associations.

In no way is it legal to reproduce, duplicate, or transmit any part of this document in either electronic means or in printed format. Recording of this publication is strictly prohibited and any storage of this document is not allowed unless with written permission from the publisher. All rights reserved.

The information provided herein is stated to be truthful and consistent, in that any liability, in terms of inattention or otherwise, by any usage or abuse of any policies, processes, or directions contained within is the solitary and utter responsibility of the recipient reader. Under no circumstances will any legal responsibility or blame be held against the publisher for any reparation, damages, or monetary loss due to the information herein, either directly or indirectly.

Respective authors own all copyrights not held by the publisher.

The information herein is offered for informational purposes solely, and is universal as so. The presentation of the information is without contract or any type of guarantee assurance. The trademarks that are used are without any consent, and the publication of the trademark is without permission or backing by the trademark owner. All trademarks and brands within this book are for clarifying purposes only and are the owned by the owners themselves, not affiliated with this document

# TABLE OF CONTENTS

Introduction ........................................................................... 5

DIY Hand Sanitizer Gel or Spray At Home ...................... 13

Homemade Hand Sanitizer .................................................. 24

When and How to Wash Your Hands ............................... 28

Guide on the correct way to use the hand sanitizers 33

Hand sanitizer tips ................................................................ 38

# INTRODUCTION

Alcohol-based hand sanitizer is easy to utilize, helpful, and frequently simple to discover. While there is a right method to utilize hand sanitizer to get the most profit by it, what's presumably increasingly significant is realizing when utilizing it may not be the best decision. Hand sanitizer can help kill microbes. However, it isn't compelling on all germs and will fail to help different substances that might be on your hands.

The Centers for Disease Control (CDC) suggests cleaning your hands with cleanser and water at whatever point conceivable (and consistently when your hands are dirty). Hand sanitizer can be utilized what's more or when washing isn't an alternative.

**Use Sanitizer When...**

You can't wash with cleanser and water

You need included protection in the wake of washing

**Try not to Use Sanitizer...**

*Hand Sanitizer Recipes*

Instead of washing with cleanser and water

At the point when your hands are noticeably grimy

At the point when you have synthetic concoctions on your hands

## How It Works

At the point when sanitizers previously turned out, there was little research demonstrating what they did and didn't do. However, that has changed. More research should be done. However, researchers are learning all the more regularly.

The active ingredient in hand sanitizers is isopropyl liquor (scouring alcohol), a comparable type of alcohol (ethanol or n-propanol), or a mix of them. Alcohols have, for some time, been known to kill organisms by dissolving their external defensive layer of proteins and disturbing their metabolism.

As indicated by the CDC, explore shows that hand sanitizer eliminates germs as successfully as washing your hands with cleanser and water—except if your hands are grimy or oily. They

*Introduction*

additionally don't expel conceivably unsafe chemicals.

Hand sanitizers likewise don't execute some regular germs cleanser, and water do take out, for example,

- Cryptosporidium
- Clostridium difficile
- Norovirus

**Bacteria and Virus Protection**

The U.S. food and Drug Administration (FDA) has made a legitimate move against some hand sanitizer organizations for making doubtful cases against salmonella, e. Coli, Ebola, rotavirus, flu, and MRSA (methicillin-resistant Staphylococcus aureus).

Simultaneously, however, contemplates are starting to recommend that alcohol-based hand sanitizers might be powerful at executing a portion of these germs. (All things considered, the organizations that cause them to seem still to pick up FDA approval for these utilizations, making any cases to this end illegal.)

*Hand Sanitizer Recipes*

**For instance:**

- A recent report on hospital-borne infections shows sanitizers may help moderate the spread of MRSA and different diseases by giving a snappy, simple, and advantageous path for human services laborers to improve their hand hygiene.

- Research distributed in 2015 presumed that alcohol-based sanitizers had the option to diminish the populaces of salmonella and E.coli.

- Concentrated hand-sanitizer use in Japan because of a flu pandemic may have stopped term paces of norovirus.

- In an examination of grade schools, hand sanitizers cut absences deficiencies because of sickness by 26% and decreased affirmed instances of disease from the profoundly infectious flu, an infection by 52%. It was, be that as it may, less viable against the influenza B virus.

- A recent report on childcare focuses found a drop in days missed due to disease when the center presented hand sanitizers and taught staff, kids, and guardians on their appropriate use.

*Introduction*

Nonetheless, it's imperative to recollect that not the entirety of the exploration is convincing. Indeed, one investigation on long healthcare services offices recommended that workers' inclination for sanitizers over cleanser and water may have added to *norovirus* outbreaks.

Besides, the nuances of a portion of these ends can be confounding. For instance, an investigation distributed in 2019 noticed that an ethanol-based hand sanitizer diminished *norovirus* contamination chance by 85% when there's transient contact with the infection. However, under high-contamination conditions, for example, those you may discover on a cruise ship or in a long term care facility, the sanitizer offered no security whatsoever.

## Does Hand Sanitizer Create Superbugs?

There have been alerts about certain antibacterial products making organisms build up protection from anti-microbials, transforming them into lethal "superbugs" (e.g., MRSA and *Clostridium difficile*). These reports originated from *triclosan,* an ingredient that was utilized in certain cleansers and hand sanitizers. The FDA prohibited the utilization of tricolsan in these products in 2019, so this worry doesn't relate to alcohol-based hand sanitizers that are presently available in the U.S.

## What to Look For

The CDC suggests sanitizers with at any rate 60% alcohol content. Most products contain somewhere in the range of 60% and 95%, yet don't accept that the higher the rates are progressively viable. To work at top productivity, these products additionally need to contain some water.

A few products available cases to disinfect your hands, however, contain too little liquor or no alcohol by any stretch of the imagination. These products will probably not offer you sufficient protection.

## Step by step instructions to Use It

At the point when hand sanitizers accomplish work, their adequacy depends on a few elements. Notwithstanding which product you use, they include:

*Introduction*

- The amount you use
- Appropriate technique
- Consistency

A few circumstances where utilization of a hand sanitizer might be proper incorporate when you're riding open transportation, have shaken hands, or contacted an animal after you've contacted a grocery cart, etc.

To utilize hand sanitizer correctly:

- Spot the suggested sum in the palm of one hand. (Peruse the producer's directions.)
- Rub your hands together, covering your whole hand, including between your fingers.
- Quit focusing on the sanitizer just once your skin is dry.

Take care to keep alcohol-based hand disinfecting gel out of the span of little youngsters, as it tends to be exceptionally hazardous whenever swallowed. The high alcohol substance can be deadly to a young child.

*Hand Sanitizer Recipes*

## When Not to Use It

Hand sanitizer ought not to be utilized rather than cleanser and water when:

- Washing is convenient
- Your hands are oily or noticeably grimy
- You have chemicals on your hands
- You may have been presented to infectious agents that aren't murdered by hand sanitizer
- You're in a high-infection situation

To keep yourself and your family sound, it's particularly essential to clean your hands after you've utilized the bathroom or arranged nourishment. Enthusiastically washing your hands with warm water and cleanser for 20 seconds is best.

# CHAPTER # 1

# DIY HAND SANITIZER GEL OR SPRAY AT HOME

If you can't discover hand sanitizers at the store, if you like to DIY your hand sanitizers, there are approaches to make them at home with household items that you most likely have.

You can include vitamin E as an optional thing. Vitamin E assists with feeding and shields your skin from the body's free radicals. You can likewise make every one without aloe Vera gel if you want to utilize a fluid splash.

## The most effective method to Make Hand Sanitizer with Vodka

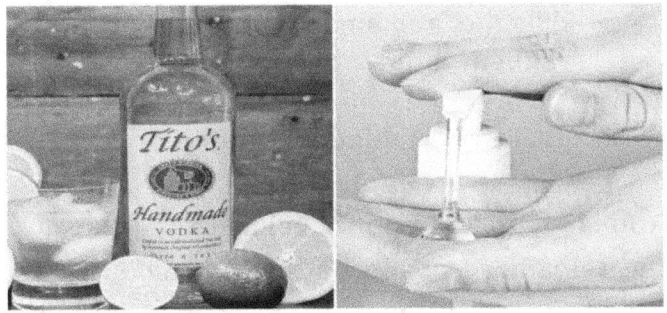

If you have a container of additional vodka lying

around at home, you can transform it into a compelling hand sanitizer to kill off harmful bacteria. Vodka has anti-microbial properties that make it a brilliant household thing for killing germs

## Here's How to Make Hand Sanitizer with Vodka:

1. Utilizing a little bottle (travel size), fill it 1/3 of the way with vodka

2. Include a couple of drops of fundamental oils of your decision (lavender oil or tea tree oil works incredibly). Note that this progression is discretionary. The essential design is to make the smell of vodka increasingly lovely.

3. Fill the remainder of the bottle with refined water

4. Shake to combine everything.

Note, if you like to utilize gel instead, you can fill the remainder of the bottle with aloe gel also. Aloe has extraordinary soothing properties that can assist with soothing sensitive skin.

*DIY Hand Sanitizer Gel or Spray At Home*

# The most effective method to Make Hand Sanitizer with Rubbing Alcohol (Isopropyl)

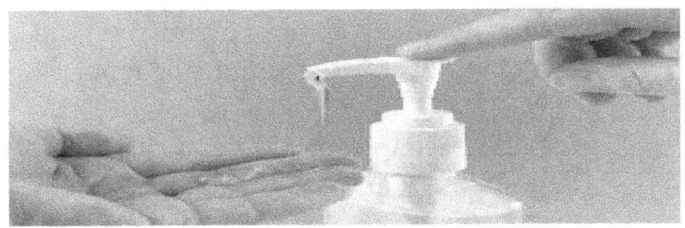

If you don't have vodka lying around at home, you can attempt to utilize rubbing alcohol. Remember that rubbing alcohol is not the same as vodka since it is lethal and can't be expended.

Before beginning, here is the thing that you have to know:

- Rubbing alcohol is normally 70% Isopropyl Alcohol by volume (ABV)

- Vodka is about 40% ABV

- Both kills bacteria (however doesn't prevent development)

This implies you don't have to use as a lot of rubbing alcohol in your hand sanitizers to accomplish the equivalent ABV.

*Hand Sanitizer Recipes*

## Here's How to Make Hand Sanitizer with Rubbing Alcohol:

1. Utilizing a small bottle (travel size), fill it 1/4 of the way with rubbing alcohol

2. Include a couple of essential oils of your decision (lavender oil or tea tree oil works extraordinarily)

3. Fill the remainder of the bottle with distilled water

4. Shake to combine everything.

Similarly, as with vodka, you can utilize aloe Vera gel rather than distilled water if you want to utilize gel overspray.

## 3. How to Make Hand Sanitizer with Essential Oils

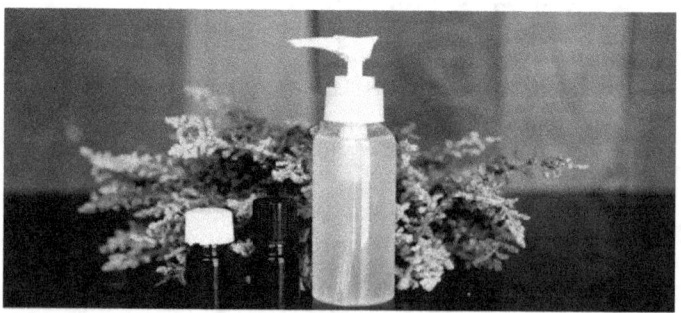

## DIY Hand Sanitizer Gel or Spray At Home

If you have sensitive skin or if you want to go to all characteristics. There is an approach to make hand sanitizers utilizing just fundamental oils and natural ingredients. Studies have demonstrated that essential oils can eliminate microorganisms, and they can give your hands a charming aroma.

Here's How to make Hand Sanitizers with Essential Oils:

1. Utilizing a small bottle (travel size) include 2 teaspoons of witch hazel.
2. Include 6 drops every one of lemon, orange, or tea tree oil.
3. Fill the container with distilled water
4. Shake to combine everything

You can utilize aloe Vera gel rather than distilled water if you like to utilize gel. Aloe is likewise incredible for diminishing inflammation and soothing your skin.

If you intend to utilize this recipe, I prescribe utilizing Handcraft Tea Tree Essential Oil. This is a 100% Pure and natural therapeutic grade oil that has been tried for its constituents just as to have no fillers, added substances, and to be undiluted. It doesn't contain chemicals, sulfates, or parabens. It is cruelty-free and created in an FDA-endorsed cGMP facility.

This oil arrives in an enormous 4oz (120ml) jar with a top-notch quality glass dropper. It is gladly bundled in the USA.

## 4.Aloe Vera Gel Alternatives for Making Hand Sanitizers

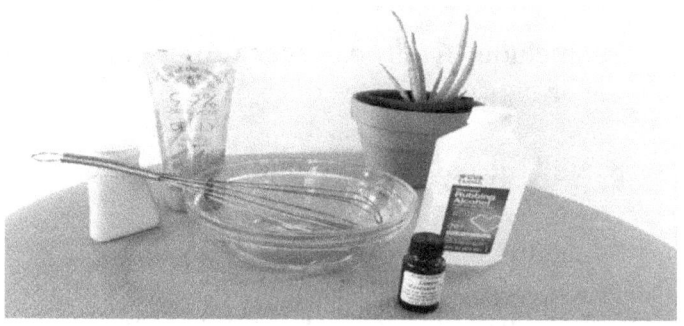

Disclaimer: To be utilized uniquely with Essential Oils Method

If you can't discover aloe vera gel, you can attempt Treatise B-glucan Water Gel. This is a top-notch calming water gel that is superb for dry

*DIY Hand Sanitizer Gel or Spray At Home*

and delicate skin. It contains an organic complex that assists with moisture skin, keep up skin ph, and strengthen your skin's unique quality.

Notable ingredients include:

- Centella Extract – assists speed with increasing skin cell creation and collagen synthesis.

- Broccoli Extract – assists with boosting defensive and detoxifying reactions in skin cells.

- Valerian Extract – serves to soothe skin.

You may likewise consider other face and skin gels like the Kala Health Max Strength Skin and Facial Gel. This gel contains unadulterated MSM (MethylsulfonylMethane), which is known as "Nature's Beauty Mineral" and is the natural type of sulfur. MSM is removed utilizing a multi-organize refining process. This gel is non-GMO, gluten-free, and allergen-free. It likewise contains aloe to help calm your skin.

MSM assists with making your skin smoother and brighter. It additionally assists with decreasing

*Hand Sanitizer Recipes*

scarcely discernible differences and wrinkles and restore collagen production.

Aquagel is another choice to attempt. This is a reasonable, water-solvent, non-irritating lubricant that is perfect with characteristic and synthetic substances. It is hypoallergenic and bacteriostatic (prevents bacteria from duplicating).

It likewise arrives in a convenient siphon bottle, which is ideal for making hand sanitizers with.

## 5.The most effective method to Make Hand Sanitizer With Glycerin

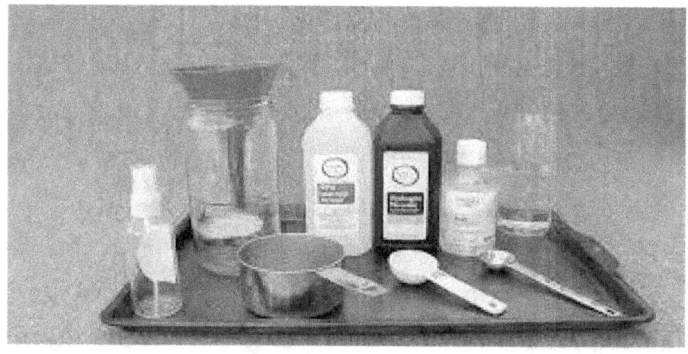

Glycerin is a three-carbon tri-alcohol humectant that is, for the most part, utilized in skincare items as a kind of moisturizing agent. In any case,

*DIY Hand Sanitizer Gel or Spray At Home*

it considers showing that utilizing glycerin can forestall the development of microscopic organisms and inactivate viruses.

Here's How to make Hand Sanitizers with Glycerin:

1. Utilizing a small bottle (travel size) includes two teaspoons of glycerin.

2. Include 1/2 teaspoon of rubbing alcohol

3. Include a couple of drops of essential oils of your decision. (like to utilize lavender oil and tea tree oil)

4. Fill the bottle with distilled water or with aloe Vera gel if you want to utilize gel rather than spray.

If you plan on utilizing this recipe, I suggest utilizing Sky Organics Vegetable Glycerin. This glycerin is USDA Organic certified, non-GMO, cold-pressed, and chemical Free. It is Hypoallergenic and effectively dissolvable in water, making it perfect for making hand sanitizers. It is likewise, odorless.

## 6.The most effective method to Make Hand

*Hand Sanitizer Recipes*

## Sanitizer with Hydrogen Peroxide

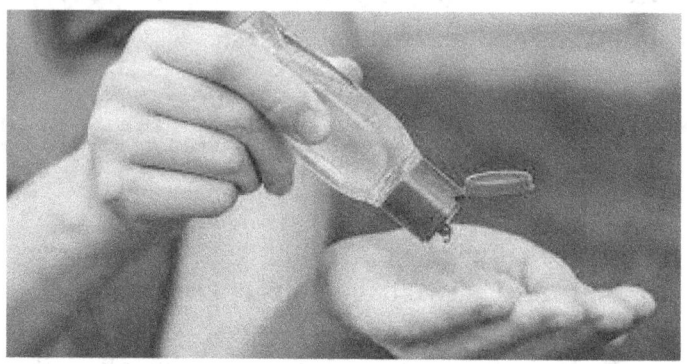

Hydrogen peroxide is comprised of a blend of hydrogen and water. It is a clear fluid that goes about as a mild antiseptic and is normally utilized on the skin to keep contaminations from minor cuts.

Here's How to make Hand Sanitizers with Hydrogen Peroxide:

1. Utilizing a little jug (travel size), fill 1/3 of the bottle with hydrogen peroxide.

2. Include a couple of drops of essential oils of your choice.

3. Fill the container with refined water or with aloe Vera gel

*DIY Hand Sanitizer Gel or Spray At Home*

4. Shake the bottle and ensure everything is mixed evenly

I find that utilizing the aloe Vera gel works better for this strategy since it assists with covering the scent fragrance of hydrogen peroxide.

# CHAPTER # 2

# HOMEMADE HAND SANITIZER

**Ingredients**

- 2-ounce spray bottle

- 5 drops nutrient E oil (discretionary, this makes for delicate hands!)

- 3 tablespoons witch hazel with aloe Vera, vodka, or 190 proof alcohol (Everclear),

- 5 drops lemon essential oil

- 5 drops orange essential oil

- 5 drops tea tree essential oil

- Distilled (or if nothing else sifted, boiled, and cooled) water

- Mark sheet, printer, and scissors

**Directions**

*Homemade Hand Sanitizer*

1. In the spray bottle, join the nutrient E oil, witch hazel, vodka or grain alcohol and essential oils. Spot the sprayer on firmly and shake well for 15-20 seconds to join.

2. Open the bottle and fill it to the top with water. Supplant sprayer, and shake again for 15-20 seconds. Done!

3. Print and stick the mark to the jug. If you don't have mark sheets kicking around, you can likewise print the name onto normal paper, and afterward, utilize clear pressing tape to cling the name to the container by utilizing the tape like an overlay over the whole name.

4. Splash generously on your hands at whatever point you feel like they need somewhat of a profound clean. Rub hands together until dry.

## Notes

**CORONAVIRUS DISCLAIMER**: This hand sanitizer is anything but a substitute for proper hand-washing. And keeping in mind that this home cure contains regularly acknowledged characteristic antiviral fixings, it has never been

## Hand Sanitizer Recipes

tried in a lab to decide it's adequacy against infections, for example, the coronavirus. The main adaptation of this hand sanitizer formula that incorporates the 60%+ alcohol content that the CDC and other wellbeing associations prescribe for hand sanitizer to appropriately murder coronavirus is the variant utilizing 190 proof grain alcohol (Everclear)— and this rendition has still not been tried for viability against coronavirus. A tried recipe that contains the correct degree of liquor can be found through the World Health Organization. As usual, check with your human services proficient before utilizing any home cure for you or your family.

**Essential oil disclaimer**: This recipe utilizes what is commonly viewed as protected essential oils, yet please remember that while regular, every single essential oil is an amazing plant intensifies that you and your family (counting your pets) may have a response to. Never utilize essential oils undiluted or take essential oils inside (weakened or undiluted) without the direction of an expert, and consistently read up about the conceivable reactions of each sort of oil before you use it. Keep away from the utilization of essential oils (diluted or undiluted) during the main trimester of pregnancy, on little infants, and anybody with serious hypersensitivities to the plants, the oils are gotten from. What's more, if you see any responses in yourself, your family, or your pets, stop utilization of your essential oil items promptly and contact medical professionals

**Utilization of high-proof grain alcohol**: Using high-proof grain alcohol (Everclear) right now be very drying on the hands.

# CHAPTER # 3

# WHEN AND HOW TO WASH YOUR HANDS

Hand washing is probably the ideal approach to shield yourself and your family from becoming ill. Realize when and how you should wash your hands to remain sound.

## Wash Your Hands Often to Stay Healthy

You can support yourself, and your friends and family remain sound by washing your hands regularly, particularly during these key occasions when you are probably going to get and spread germs:

- Previously, during, and in the wake of getting ready nourishment
- Before eating nourishment
- When thinking about somebody at home who is wiped out with heaving or
- Vomiting and diarrhea

*When and How to Wash Your Hands*

- When treating a cut or wound
- After utilizing the toilet
- After switching diapers or tidying up a kid who has utilized the toilet
- After cleaning out your nose, coughing, or sneezing
- After contacting an animal, animal feed, or animal waste
- After dealing with pet nourishment or pet treats
- After contacting garbage

## Follow Five Steps to Wash Your Hands the Right Way

Washing your hands is simple, and it's one of the best approaches to forestall the spread of germs. Clean hands can prevent germs from spreading, starting with one individual then onto the next and all through a whole community—from your home and work environment to childcare offices and hospitals.

Follow these five stages without fail.

*Hand Sanitizer Recipes*

1. Wet your hands with perfect, running water (warm or cold), turn off the tap, and apply cleanser.

2. Foam your hands by scouring them together with the cleanser. Foam the backs of your hands, between your fingers, and under your nails.

3. Scour your hands for in any event 20 seconds. Need a clock? Murmur, the "Cheerful Birthday" melody from start to finish twice.

4. Wash your hands thoroughly under perfect, running water.

5. Dry your hands utilizing a perfect towel or air dry them.

## Use Hand Sanitizer When You Can't Use Soap and Water

You can utilize an alcohol-based hand sanitizer that contains in any event 60% liquor if cleanser and water are not accessible.

Washing hands with cleanser and water are the

*When and How to Wash Your Hands*

ideal approach to dispose of germs by and large. If soap and water are not promptly accessible, you can utilize a liquor based hand sanitizer that contains at any rate 60% alcohol. You can tell if the sanitizer contains in any event 60% alcohol by taking a product label.

Sanitizers can rapidly diminish the number of germs on hands as a rule. Nonetheless,

- Sanitizers don't dispose of a wide range of germs.

- Hand sanitizers may not be as powerful when hands are obviously filthy or oily.

- Hand sanitizers probably won't expel harmful chemicals from hands like pesticides and overwhelming metals.

**Caution!** Swallowing alcohol-based hand sanitizers can cause liquor harming if more than several significant pieces are swallowed. Keep it far from little youngsters and direct their utilization. Learn increasingly here.

## The most effective method to utilize hand sanitizer

*Hand Sanitizer Recipes*

- Apply the gel item to the palm of one hand (read the name to get familiar with the right amount).

- Rub your hands together.

- Rub the gel over all the surfaces of your hands and fingers until your hands are dry. This should take around 20 seconds.

New Handwashing Campaign: Life is better with Clean Hands

To observe Global Handwashing Day on October 15, CDC has propelled the Life is Better with Clean Hands crusade. This campaign urges grown-ups to make handwashing some portion of their regular day to day existence and urges guardians to wash their hands to set a genuine model for their children.

# CHAPTER # 4

# GUIDE ON THE CORRECT WAY TO USE THE HAND SANITIZERS

CDC suggests washing hands with cleanser and water at whatever point conceivable because hand washing diminishes the measures of a wide range of germs and synthetic compounds on hands. In any case, if cleanser and water are not accessible, utilizing a hand sanitizer with, at any rate, 60% alcohol can assist you with abstaining from becoming ill and spreading germs to other people. The direction for compelling hand washing and utilization of hand sanitizer in community settings was created dependent on information from various investigations.

Alcohol-based hand sanitizers can rapidly lessen the number of organisms on hands in certain circumstances, yet sanitizers don't dispense with a wide range of germs.

Why? Cleanser and water are more successful than hand sanitizers at expelling particular sorts of germs, like Cryptosporidium, norovirus, and

*Hand Sanitizer Recipes*

Clostridium difficile. Even though liquor based hand sanitizers can inactivate numerous sorts of microorganisms viably when utilized effectively, individuals may not utilize a huge enough volume of the sanitizers or may clear it off before it has dried.

**Hand sanitizers may not be as powerful when hands are unmistakably dirty or greasy.**

**Why**? Numerous examinations show that hand sanitizers function admirably in clinical settings like emergency clinics, where hands come into contact with germs; however, for the most part, they are not vigorously grimy or oily. A few pieces of information additionally show that hand sanitizers may function admirably against particular sorts of germs on somewhat dirty hands. Nonetheless, hands may turn out to be extremely oily or ruined in network settings, for example, after individuals handle nourishment, play sports, work in the nursery, or go outdoors or angling. At the point when hands are vigorously filthy or oily, hand sanitizers may not function admirably. Handwashing with cleanser and water is suggested in such conditions.

*Guide on the correct way to use sanitizers*

**Hand sanitizers probably won't expel harmful chemicals, similar to pesticides and overwhelming metals, from hands.**

**Why?** Although few any investigations have been led, hand sanitizers presumably can't expel or inactivate numerous kinds of unsafe synthetic concoctions. In one examination, individuals who announced utilizing hand sanitizer to clean hands had expanded degrees of pesticides in their bodies. If hands have contacted harmful chemicals, wash cautiously with cleanser and water (or as coordinated by a toxic substance control focus).

**If cleanser and water are not accessible, utilize a liquor based hand sanitizer that contains if 60% alcohol.**

**W**hy? Numerous examinations have discovered that sanitizers with a liquor fixation between 60–95% are more compelling at eliminating germs than those with a lower liquor focus or non-alcohol based hand sanitizers. Hand sanitizers without 60-95% liquor 1) may not work similarly well for some kinds of germs, and 2) only lessen the development of germs instead of killing them

*Hand Sanitizer Recipes*

by and large.

**When utilizing hand sanitizer, apply the item to the palm of one hand (read the name to get familiar with the right sum) and rub the item everywhere throughout the surfaces of your hands until your hands are dry.**

Why? The means for hand sanitizer use depend on an improved technique prescribed by the CDC. Training individuals to cover all surfaces of two hands with hand sanitizer has been found to give comparable purification viability as giving definite strides to focusing close by sanitizer.

**Swallowing alcohol-based hand sanitizers can cause liquor poisoning.**

Why? Ethyl liquor (ethanol) - based hand sanitizers are sheltered when utilized as coordinated, yet they can cause liquor harming if individual swallows over a few pieces.

From 2011 – 2015, U.S. poison control focuses got almost 85,000 calls about hand sanitizer exposures among youngsters. Kids might

*Guide on the correct way to use sanitizers*

probably swallow hand sanitizers that are scented, brilliantly hued, or alluringly bundled. Hand sanitizers ought to be put away out of the compass of little youngsters and ought to be utilized with adult supervision. Child-resistant tops could likewise help diminish hand sanitizer-related poisonings among small kids. Older youngsters and grown-ups may intentionally swallow hand sanitizers to get alcoholics.

# CHAPTER # 5

# HAND SANITIZER TIPS

Glance around and will undoubtedly observe an alcohol-based hand sanitizer someplace close by. They're wherever nowadays - in washrooms, in kitchens, dangling from ropes appended to children's rucksacks and rising out of ladies' backpacks, roosted on the dividers of school cafeterias and along with the hall hospitals of the and nursing homes.

There are loads of acceptable, logically demonstrated reasons why alcohol-based hand sanitizers are all over the place:

- At the point when you're not ready to wash your hands, hand sanitizers offer a protected and compelling substitute for a soap-and-water scrub.

- Gels containing at any rate 60% germ-killing alcohol can shield you and your family from the bugs that cause colds and gastrointestinal infections.

*Hand sanitizer tips*

- Social insurance laborers in hospitals and other medicinal services settings utilize the alcohol-based hand gels. At the point when their hands are not unmistakably dirty, the alcohol-based sanitizers are more successful than ordinary hand-washing or purifying with an antibacterial cleanser.

However, before you go hurl out all the bars of soap in the house, consider these hand sanitizer realities:

- **Hand sanitizers don't wipe off noticeable dirt.** They're intended to eliminate germs, yet if you can see soil, grime, blood, or whatever else, you have to wash with cleanser and water.

- **Not all sanitizers viably eliminate germs.** Assess the name cautiously. Verify that the sanitizer contains a convergence of 60% to 95% ethanol (ethyl liquor) or isopropanol (isopropyl liquor). Anything short of 60% won't viably eliminate germs. Watch for these below average plans in the deal canister or at dollar stores.

*Hand Sanitizer Recipes*

- **Sanitizers can be toxic**. These products contain significant levels of liquor, and some come in tantalizingly scented varieties. Kids can be enticed to taste the gel. A tiny lick at their cleaned skin shouldn't do any harm, yet ingesting an excessive amount of can cause alcohol poisoning. For tidiness and accommodation, numerous guardians are sending scaled-down jugs of sanitizer to class with their little youngsters. Some more up to date rucksack models even accompany a connection for them! Children may think of it as a toy - or a treat - and share it with companions. Show your children sanitizer security and urge them to utilize the product appropriately and just when completely essential.

- **The ingredients can bother**. Alcohol is drying to the skin, and included scents may trigger unfavorably susceptible reactions and irritations. Many hand sanitizers contain creams to balance the drying impact.

- Sanitizers must be utilized appropriately

*Hand sanitizer tips*

to work adequately. To appropriately apply hand sanitizers, you have to evacuate any rings initially. Utilize a dime-sized drop of the gel and rub your hands together, palm to palm. At that point, utilize the palm of one hand to rub the gel into the rear of the other hand and among fingers, and the other way around. Remember to rub around the thumbs, also. Keep on scouring the gel into your hands until they feel dry, generally for at any rate 15 to 30 seconds. You shouldn't require a towel to get dry.

## Things You Don't Know About Hand Sanitizers, 3 Tips to Buy It Right

You can't fight a thought with rationale. That is my decision in the wake of viewing my 70-year-old mother fixate close by sanitizer.

My mother showed me how to set aside cash by cutting coupons and checking my pockets for spare change. However, she has no issue burning through $3 for a little jug of hand sanitizer that she conveys wherever in her handbag. Also, no measure of research on this point will adjust her perspective or her ways of managing money.

*Hand Sanitizer Recipes*

"Mother, you realize that stuff doesn't function just as you might suspect it does, right?" I ask her once while we were sitting in an eatery, where I was getting her Mother's Day supper.

"Indeed, it's superior to nothing," she answered, squirting some on her hands from her small jug.

"Not comparable to washing our hands, which we can do by going over yonder," I stated, highlighting the bathrooms.

"Dear, if this didn't work, at that point, for what reason would they sell such an extensive amount it?" she asked, holding out the modest jug so she could squirt some in my grasp.

In light of a legitimate concern for family harmony, I scoured a portion of the stuff on my hands. At that point, I pardoned myself and went to wash my hands in the men's room.

My mother is directly around a certain something: Americans do purchase a great deal of hand sanitizer – $117 million worth consistently – even though there's sparse proof they work how we figure they do…

*Hand sanitizer tips*

**WE THINK** hand sanitizer executes "99.9 percent of germs" when we use them.

**WE KNOW** that it is just under lab conditions. "If you take this present reality model where individuals are not washing their hands consistently and all the soil and grime isn't removed their hands preceding utilizing a hand sanitizer, the genuine viability of the sanitizer is going to diminish, " Indiana University microbiologist Jason Tetro gave an account of his school's podcast. "It's anyplace somewhere in the range of 40 and 60 percent compelling."

**WE THINK** all hand sanitizers are the equivalent.

**WE KNOW** hand sanitizers with under 60 percent ethyl or isopropyl liquor are slightly below average at eliminating germs – even though a few brands available contain just 40 percent. "Indeed, utilizing a liquor sanitizer with just 40 percent liquor probably won't lessen microorganisms on your hands by any means.

**WE THINK** hand sanitizer keeps our hands clean for a considerable length of time.

**WE KNOW** them a minute ago. "The main items

*Hand Sanitizer Recipes*

available today dispense with germs on contact yet work for as meager as two minutes," says another study that asked Americans to what extent they think their hand sanitizer last. The outcomes? "58 percent of the 1,007 people surveyed said they accept their hand sanitizer saves germs under control for an hour or more." Claim the survey released not long ago.

Most telling was this outcome: "Of those Americans who use hand sanitizers, 71 percent said they use them for significant serenity." She describes my mother, consummately.

Why every one of these confusions? Since promoting works superior to inquire about. If that you go to the Purell site, you'll see an adorable young man cleaning out his nose. If you look into thorough scholarly research about the adequacy of hand sanitizer, you get a page without any photos and a title like, "A Randomized, Controlled Trial of a Multifaceted Intervention Including Alcohol-Based Hand Sanitizer and Hand-Hygiene Education to Reduce Illness Transmission in the Home."

Coincidentally, those examinations do uncover one significant truth: While washing your hands

*Hand sanitizer tips*

is ideal, hand sanitizer accomplishes work on the off chance that you keep its viability in context. In light of that, here are three hints for purchasing the stuff...

**Read the label:** "Check the bottle for dynamic ingredients," Columbia teacher Elaine Larson revealed to The New York Times. "It may state ethyl liquor, ethanol, isopropanol or some other variety, and those are on the whole fine. However, ensure that whichever of those alcohols is recorded, its fixation is somewhere in the range of 60 and 95 percent. Not as much as that isn't sufficient."

**Utilize a great deal**: You previously purchased the stuff, so don't hold back on utilizing it now. "What amount of gel would it be advisable for you to utilize? Enough to continue scouring for 20 seconds without drying totally," prescribes Dr. Benabio. "If the alcohol vanishes in under 15 seconds, at that point, you're not utilizing enough."

**Purchase in bulk and online**: At least my mom purchases enormous top off bottles of hand sanitizer to top off her bottles. Alas, she doesn't shop on the web, where costs are even lower.

*Hand Sanitizer Recipes*

Another motivation to stock up Prices goes up when the request does. So, for example, a year ago, during flu season, hand sanitizer took off the racks, up 70 percent during October 2009 from a similar period the prior year. So like whatever else, stock up when the request is down.

**BENEFITS OF HAND SANITIZER**

You realize you have to keep your hands clean. As much as your hands serve you, they additionally put germs in contact with your mouth, eyes, nose, and numerous different pieces of your body. We trust you're as of now washing your hands with cleanser and warm water on various occasions a day, as that is the ideal approach to clean them, however, another commendable option is hand sanitizer. If you haven't just made this germ-fighter a staple on your shopping show, you might need to do as such after finding out about the advantages of hand sanitizer

**Advantage 1: CLEANLINESS**

This shouldn't come as quite a bit of a surprise. One of the first advantages of hand sanitizer is only that: It cleans. These products were intended to eliminate germs, and they take care

*Hand sanitizer tips*

of business. At the point when utilized appropriately, hand sanitizers can kill 99.9% of the germs on your hands. The CDC prescribes washing your hands whenever you're around nourishment (getting ready it or eating it), animals, trash, and more. At the point when you end up in these circumstances, hand sanitizer is the ideal expansion to (or infrequent swap for) washing your hands with soap and water.

## Advantage 2: PORTABILITY

Last time we checked, you can't take a sink in a hurry. In those circumstances where you have to wash your hands, there isn't continually going to be cleanser and water accessible. You can slip a little container of hand sanitizer in your glove compartment, a tote, or even your pocket for circumstances where you should wash your hands; however, either can't discover a sink or hang tight for one is badly designed (think long queues or far away bathrooms). Its ideal for when you're snatching a nibble at a game or have recently left an open space, similar to the supermarket.

## Advantage 3: GREAT FOR GROUP SETTINGS

*Hand Sanitizer Recipes*

At the workplace, in the study hall, or any space with heaps of pedestrian activity, germs spread rapidly. Also, regardless of whether you're not preparing to eat or taking out the trash, others' germs can influence you (particularly nearby other people). That is the reason having hand sanitizer accessible is perfect for bunch settings. Instructors, students, and office laborers can eliminate germs intermittently for the day without leaving their study hall or work area, and exercise center goers can utilize a squirt of hand sanitizer before jumping on the following workout machine.

**Advantage 4: LESS RISK FOR DISEASE**

Particularly during flu season, limiting your presentation to others' germs is vital for your wellbeing. At the point when you pause for a minute to disinfect your hands a couple of times for the day, you diminish your odds of becoming ill. Indeed, even an active excursion to a companion's home or the store can open you to germs that could cause a chilly, the flu, or different diseases, so keeping your hands as perfect as conceivable is significant.

**Advantage 5: SOFTER-FEELING HANDS**

*Hand sanitizer tips*

This may be one of the most astonishing advantages of hand sanitizer. However, it isn't unrealistic. Hand sanitizers that don't contain alcohol can improve the surface of the skin on your hands (note that hand sanitizers with alcohol won't have this impact). Some hand sanitizers contain emollients that relax your skin, giving you more pleasant looking and smoother hands. You'll certainly see a distinction in how saturated your skin feels and looks. Stay away from hand sanitizers that contain alcohol, as they wash away the skin's common oils and can make the skin break, which in turn makes a passage point for bacteria.

There are numerous advantages of hand sanitizer, from fighting germs proficiently to fighting them helpfully (and in any event, improving your skin). No, ifs, ands or buts, utilizing this germ-fighting product consistently for the day will support your cleanliness and your wellbeing regardless of where life takes you.

**Limitations:**

- Not all hand sanitizers are made similarly. Check the container for active ingredients. The alcohol content might be as ethyl

*Hand Sanitizer Recipes*

> alcohol, ethanol, or isopropanol. Those are satisfactory types of alcohol. Be sure that regardless of which sort of alcohol is recorded, its fixation is somewhere in the range of 60 and 95 percent. Am alcohol content of under 60 percent isn't sufficient to be viable.

- Alcohol doesn't slice through the grime. All earth, blood, and soil must be cleaned or washed away first if the alcohol in the sanitizer is to be successful. In such cases, hand-washing with cleanser and water is exhorted.

- Hand sanitizers are not cleaning experts and are not implied as a swap for soap and water, yet as a reciprocal propensity. Sanitizers are best when utilized related to persevering hand-washing.

The utilization of hand sanitizers is a habit that can help keep all of us presented to fewer germs, and in this manner may diminish our chance of illness. Regardless of whether you are on the play area, utilizing another person's computer, or visiting a companion in the emergency clinic, set aside the effort to rub some on your hands. It is a simple advance toward a healthy winter season.

www.ingramcontent.com/pod-product-compliance
Lightning Source LLC
Chambersburg PA
CBHW071124240526
45465CB00023B/804